Fight Back Against Sciatica

A Comprehensive Guide to Sciatica Causes, Exercises & Home Treatment

Introduction

If you've ever experienced sciatic pain, you will never forget it. From the pins and needles feeling of numbness to stabbing pains, this pain can be simply annoying or excruciating.

In this article, we will explain how sciatic pain occurs, how it is diagnosed and what can be done to ease the pain. You don't need to feel like a hostage to sciatic pain, because most people can experience relief without surgery.

There are ways you can fight back against sciatica, and we will present you with the best ways to battle this pain. From medications to stretching and yoga, and even into herbal medications, we will give you new weapons in the fight against sciatic pain.

The information herein is offered for informational purposes solely, and is universal as so. The presentation of the information is without contract or any type of guarantee assurance.

The trademarks that are used are without any consent, and the publication of the trademark is without permission or backing by the trademark owner. All trademarks and brands within this book are for clarifying purposes only and are the owned by the owners themselves, not affiliated with this document.

Table of Contents

What is Sciatica?

Sciatica is at its core a symptom of physical issues taking place within the body. It is mainly seen as leg pain, varying from what feels like bad cramps in the leg, to shooting, excruciating pain that makes sitting or standing almost impossible.

Sciatica pain may become worse when you cough or sneeze. It can come on gradually or occur more suddenly. You may feel tingling or burning, or numbness or weakness in your leg. Occasionally it will extend to the toes. The pain may make it difficult to move your foot and toes or bend your knee.

How do physicians diagnose sciatica?

To determine the cause of your sciatica, your physician will obtain a full medical history from you, including reviewing your symptoms. A physical examination will help him in diagnosing sciatica and in determining the cause.

One of the tests he may perform is the straight-leg-raise exam. In this test, you will lie flat on your back with your legs straight out. He will raise each leg slowly and note the elevation of the leg when you start to feel pain. This exam is helpful in pinpointing the nerves that are affected, and in determining if you have a disc problem in your back.

Other tests may be used to look for other sciatic pain causes. Depending on what is found, your primary care physician or specialist may recommend more testing. These tests may include:

- A myelogram, which uses dye injected between vertebrae to see if a disc or vertebra is causing your pain

- A nerve conduction velocity study or electromyography, to see how well your body's electrical impulses travel through your sciatic nerve

- A magnetic resonance imaging (MRI) scan or CAT scan to create clear images of your back structures

- An X-ray that looks for spinal fractures

Most patients, however, can be successfully treated without more testing being done.

How is sciatica treated?

The goal in sciatica treatment is increasing mobility and decreasing pain. This will most often include some limited rest, medications, then physical therapy and exercise. The medications are helpful in treating inflammation and pain.

- **Physical Therapy**

  The goal in this type of therapy is to find movements done in exercise that will decrease sciatic pain when it reduces nerve pressure. Exercise programs usually include stretching and other exercises that will improve muscle tightness and flexibility, and aerobic exercise, like walking.

- **Injections in the Spine**

  Injections of anti-inflammatory medications into your lower back can help in reducing inflammation and swelling of nerve roots, which gives you increased mobility.

- **Medications**

  Anti-inflammatory and pain drugs will help in relieving stiffness and pain, which will allow you to exercise and become more mobile. There are many over-the-counter medications in the class of non-steroidal anti-inflammatory medicines (NSAIDs) that may help, including naproxen (Aleve), aspirin and ibuprofen (Advil, Motrin)

  Muscle relaxants like Flexeril may also be prescribed, to help in relieving muscle spasm discomfort. These are not as often used in elderly patients, since they can cause confusion. Prescription medications for pain may also be used in treatment, depending on your pain level.

- **Surgery**

  Surgery is necessary if you do not respond to more conservative treatment methods, if you experience severe pain or have progressing symptoms.

  Types of surgery used include:

  Laminectomy — In this procedure, the tissues causing pressure are removed.

  Microdiscectomy — In this procedure, herniated disc fragments are removed.

- **Acupuncture and Yoga**

  These treatment modalities are sometimes used to improve sciatic pain. Massage may be helpful in alleviating muscle spasms. Biofeedback may relieve stress and manage pain, helping you cope with your pain. These are often called alternative therapies used to fight sciatica.

What are some complications of sciatica?

Lasting, ongoing pain may occur if sciatica goes untreated. If there is severe injury involving a pinched nerve, you may develop chronic weakness in the muscles of your leg or foot.

What can sciatica sufferers expect in their prognosis?

Sciatic pain will often ease with rest and time. Most people diagnosed with sciatica will recover without the need for surgery. Roughly 50% of patients with sciatica recover from episodes of pain or inflammation within about six weeks.

Can you prevent sciatica?

Many sciatica sources aren't preventable, including accidental falls, pregnancy-induced back strain and degenerative disc disease.

Although you cannot prevent all sciatica events, you can reduce your risk and protect your back:

- Avoid sitting for long periods of time.

- Use proper posture when you sit, stand and sleep. This will help in relieving lower back pressure.

- Exercise on a regular basis to strengthen your abdominal and back muscles, which support the spine.

- Stop or avoid smoking cigarettes, as this promotes the degeneration of discs.

- Practice proper techniques when you lift. Lift with a straight back, using your legs and hips to lift. Use this method even when lifting light objects.

What Causes Sciatica?

When you discuss sciatica, understanding the medical cause of symptoms is vital, since treatments focus on the root cause of pain.

The most commonly seen causes of sciatica include;

- **Degenerative Disc Disease**

    The degeneration of spinal discs happens naturally as you age, but if you have one or more discs in your lower back that have degenerated, this can irritate the roots of nerves, causing sciatic pain.

    This is diagnosed when weakened discs result in too high a level of micro-motion at this level. Inflammatory proteins from within the disc are exposed, irritating the area's nerve roots.

- **Lumbar Herniated Disc**

    Herniated discs occur when the inner core of discs herniates, or leaks out, through the outer core. This irritates the nerve root.

    Herniated discs are sometimes called pinched nerves, protruding discs, bulging discs, ruptured discs or slipped discs. The most common symptom of lumbar herniated discs is sciatica.

- **Lumbar Spinal Stenosis**

  This condition causes sciatica on a frequent basis, since it causes the spinal canal to narrow. This is related to the natural aging of the spine, and is most common in people over 60 years of age.

  It usually results from a combination of bulging discs, soft tissue overgrowth or facet joint enlargement, causing pain due to pressure on the nerve roots.

- **Isthmic Spondylolisthesis**

  This wordy condition occurs when small stress fractures allow a vertebral body to slip on another one.

  When this occurs, the fracture, collapse of disc space and the slipping forward of the vertebral body can pinch a nerve and thus cause sciatica.

- **Sacroiliac Joint Dysfunction**

  This condition occurs when the sacroiliac joint becomes irritated. It is found at the base of the spine. This may irritate your L5 nerve, lying atop the sacroiliac joint, which causes pain like sciatica.

- **Piriformis Syndrome**

  The piriformis is a deep, small hip rotator that is used when your thigh is turned out. It abducts your thigh (taking it out to the side) when you flex your hip and extends your hip when you are walking.

In some cases, your sciatic nerve may become irritated where it runs beneath the piriformis buttock muscle. If this muscle punches or irritates a nerve root and compromises your sciatic nerve, it can cause the same type of pain as sciatica.

This condition is not true sciatica, but the pain in the leg may feel much the same as nerve-irritation sciatica.

If your problem is in the piriformis, you may experience pins and needles and pain in the outer calf that may extend to the point between your fourth and little toes. You may also experience a burning sensation in the back of your calf and thigh and stiffness in the legs.

With piriformis syndrome, it may become difficult for you to walk on your toes or heels. You may feel pain when you sit, and a tingling in the back area of the thigh. Sometimes this pain is relieved when you stand, but you may still have numbness in your toes even when you are standing.

How Sciatica can Cause Back or Leg Pain

The symptoms you experience with sciatica, like weakness, tingling, nerve pain or numbness, may be different from those experienced by others. The pain may be primarily in the calf, thigh or buttock.

Sciatic Nerve Pain Types

Your symptoms and pain can often be traced to the point where the irritated or injured nerve originates in your lower back. Common symptoms may include:

- **Sciatica from the S1 nerve root**

  Sciatica symptoms that originate at this level, at the bottom of your spine, may include difficulty in walking on your tiptoes, or in raising your heel, due to weakness. You may also experience numbness or pain to the outside of your foot.

- **Sciatica from the L5 nerve root**

  If this segment of the nerve root is affected, you may experience weakness when you extend your big toe, and sometimes in your ankle, as well.

  The symptoms of sciatica that originates at this lower back level may include numbness or pain on the top of your foot, especially in the webbing between your big toe and your second toe.

- **Sciatica from the L4 nerve root**

  Symptoms of sciatica that stems from this area in the spine can include numbness or pain to your lower medial leg and foot, including the inability to walk on your heels.

What is the difference between sciatic and referred pain?

Sciatica is commonly used in the indication of any pain that is radiating into your leg. If this is caused by the sciatic nerve, this would be the correct terminology.

If your pain is referred from a joint to the leg, also known as referred pain, then it is not technically sciatica.

Referred pain from joint problems like arthritis can cause pain in the legs that feels like sciatica, and this is actually found more commonly than true sciatica.

The range of sciatica symptoms is wide, and the severity and type of pain you experience depends on the condition that causes your symptoms.

Fighting Sciatica with Stretches

In many cases of sciatic pain, a controlled and progressive program of exercise tailored to the underlying cause of the pain is an important part of your treatment program. These specific exercises have two purposes:

- Reduction of near term sciatic pain

- Providing of conditioning to aid in the prevention of future pain recurrences

The specific exercises will usually be prescribed by a certified athletic trainer, physical medicine and rehabilitation physician, chiropractor or physical therapist. They will also teach you how the exercises should be performed.

It seems a bit counterintuitive, but exercise is often more useful than bed rest for reliving your sciatic pain. After flare-ups, you may rest for one or two days, but after that, inactivity may worsen your pain.

Without movement and stretching exercise, your spinal structures and back muscles will become less able to provide support for your back. Weakening and de-conditioning may lead to strain and injury of the back, causing more pain.

Additionally, stretching exercises help in spinal disc health. Movement will help in the exchange of fluids and nutrients in the discs, keeping them healthy and helping in the prevention of more sciatic nerve pressure.

What do sciatica stretching exercise programs include?

The proper stretching exercises will help to increase the strength of your core muscles. They will strengthen the muscles in your back and abdomen, to help in providing more back support. Stretching exercises for people with sciatica will target the muscles that can cause pain when they are inflexible and tight. If you can stick to a program of regular, gentle stretching and strengthening exercises, you will recover more speedily from flare ups and you'll be less likely to have pain in the future.

Most stretching exercise programs are tailored so that they will address the main underlying cause of your sciatic pain. You can worsen your sciatic pain if you do the wrong types of exercise, so be sure you have an accurate diagnosis before you start a stretching exercise program.

Types of Sciatica Stretching Exercises

Sciatic pain starts from the irritation or pressure on your sciatic nerve. This nerve begins at the lower spine, on both sides. It runs through the buttocks and pelvic area, down the back of your thighs. This nerve splits right at the knee, and the branches extend down to your feet. Pain may stretch along this body route and it can be achy and mild or burning and sharp. Pins and needles and numbness often accompany sciatica.

If you stay in a single position for a long time, whether standing or sitting, sciatica pain usually worsens. It concentrates the pressure on the sciatic nerve and causes stressed-out muscles to become tighter. Stretching helps relax your muscles and relieves pain. It will also be a suitable warm-up for exercises designed for strengthening. Core exercise and stretching are helpful in preventing future episodes of pain, if you do them on a regular basis.

Stretches that work best to relieve sciatica pain

While working on stretching, be sure to breathe normally. Holding your breath may counteract the stretching's relaxing effect on your muscles. Do not stretch to the point that it causes you pain. Check with your physician to find out which stretching exercises will be best for your case of sciatica. Maintain a proper body position when you are stretching.

In many stretching exercises, you will start by lying on your back, supporting your neck and head. A rolled towel under your neck works well for this support.

Stretches for your Back Muscles

Lie on your back with your knees bent and your feet firm and flat on the floor. Pull your left leg towards your chest, slowly and gently. Grasp this leg with both of your hands, below and in front of your knee. Hold it there for 20 seconds and then relax. Repeat this stretch five times on each leg.

Stand with your feet a bit apart and your palms near the back of the waist atop your buttocks. Your fingers should be pointed downward. Then push your pelvis and hips slightly forward, bending the rest of your body backward. Simultaneously, bend your neck back and look up toward the ceiling. Relax and then repeat this five to ten times.

Stretch Video: https://youtu.be/H0NW3TnAT3Y

30 Minute Sciatica Stretch Video:
https://youtu.be/pyFNz8zJSdw

Stretches for the Piriformis

Bending your legs at a 45-degree angle brings your feet so they're flat on the floor. Lift your left leg high enough to place your left ankle on the right knee. Grab the left knee and pull it across your upper body in a gentle way, towards your right shoulder, until you feel your buttocks and hips stretching. Hold this position for 15 to 30 seconds and then return your left foot back to the floor. Lie and relax and then repeat the stretch with the opposite leg. Repeat this stretch two to four times, alternating the legs.

Stretch Video: https://youtu.be/CcHVBsxmJXA

Stretch Video: https://youtu.be/dl474z1bhnk

Stretches for the Hamstring

While lying on your back and bending both knees, straighten your left leg and relax it upon the floor. Your other knee should be bent at a 45 degree angle with your right foot flat on the floor. Next, place both of your hands behind your left thigh, close to the knee. If you can't reach it without help, you can use a towel, which increases your reach.

Then straighten the knee slowly while you flex your foot, and try to get the sole of that foot to face up to the ceiling. You will feel a stretching on the back of the thigh. When you feel this, hold the position for 10 seconds. Gradually work your way up on both legs until you can hold it for 20 to 30 seconds.

Video: https://youtu.be/C-wiOqYcxoI

Video 2: https://youtu.be/LZ32ho5edvo

Why You Should Stretch Your Hip Flexors

Hip flexors are an important part of using your joints properly, to avoid pain. Most people do have fairly tight hips, but they can be loosened, to break the cycle of inflexibility and stiffness that can result in pain. Stretching will cause your hip flexors to become more flexible. It's not difficult to stretch your hips.

These muscles are very important in:

- Stabilizing your lower body

- Moving your legs from front to back and side to side

- Pulling the knees upward

- Flexing the trunk forward

- Flexing the hip joint

Tight hip flexors will have a negative impact on the results of your workouts. Strong, flexible hip flexors will be helpful in getting better results from abdominal exercise.

Tightness in the hips can be found in people with anterior pelvic tilt, where the buttocks stick out more than they should. This is bad for your posture and can add to back pain. Becoming more flexible in the hips will aid in correcting anterior pelvic tilt, particularly when you combine them with core work, for better posture.

Before you stretch your hip flexors, they need to be warm. Once you're ready for active stretching, here are some of the specific exercises that work best in stretching the hip flexors.

- The happy baby pose has you flat on your back. Lift your legs until you can grab your feet at the sides. Hold for 10 to 20 seconds.

- The butterfly stretch works well to open up your hips. Sit upright on the floor with your legs in front of you. Then bend them in until your feet touch and hold your ankles with your hands.

- The head to knee stretch is similar to stretches found in yoga. Sit upright on the floor with your legs in front of you. Pull one leg back until the foot is touching the inside of your other leg, near your crotch. Then lay your head on the knee of your straight leg and reach with your arms and hands to grasp your outstretched foot.

Yoga Stretches to Fight Sciatica

Sciatica has been causing pain for many years, and some rather imaginative remedies have been tried to soothe the pain, from hot coals and leeches to injections and creams.

The Journal of Neurosurgery in 2005 estimated that over 5% of the US adult population suffers from some type of sciatic pain. Over your lifetime, there can be as high as a 40% chance that you will experience sciatic pain at some point. The good news is, a targeted and mindful yoga session uses stretches that help in overcoming the pain.

How yoga stretching helps to relieve sciatic pain

If your sciatic pain is caused by a bulging or herniated disc, it may benefit you to pursue yoga stretching that progresses slowly from gentle poses to those that are more foundational in nature. Speak with your primary care physician to ensure that the stretching you are doing will benefit you and not exacerbate your condition.

Poses like the down-ward facing dog and standing poses will lengthen, strengthen and align your lower back. Herniated discs don't always require surgery, so yoga will be helpful in managing and reducing the problems brought about by herniation, and it may even reduce that herniation.

If your sciatica is the result of a tight, short piriformis, stretching that muscle will ease your pain. Use a gentle approach, and do not overwork the piriformis, or you may experience spasms or buttock pain.

The Standing Twist

This is a milder version of some other yoga stretches, which will help the muscles in your back. It will bring your thigh into internal rotation. To do this exercise, place a chair flat against a wall. Stand with your right side closest to the wall to start stretching of the right hip. Place your right foot atop the chair, and bend your knee at about 90 degrees. Your left leg should remain straight.

Steady yourself by placing the right hand against the wall. Lift up your left heel, putting your weight on the mounds of your toes. Turn your body in the direction of the wall. Exhale and lower your left heel back onto the floor, but maintain the twist you have created. Allow your right hip now to descend, while keeping your hips level. Hold this position for several breaths.

Video: https://youtu.be/HQEFH1gGg1g

The Simple Seated Twist

In this stretch, your upper body will turn toward your upright knee. Help your upper body in turning completely by placing your left hand behind you, on the floor. Hold your left knee securely with the right hand. Make sure to keep your chest lifted and your lower back in its natural curve. When you inhale, expand and lengthen. When you exhale, twist gently, without allowing your back to become rounded.

Next, the action upon the piriformis can be deepened by releasing groin tightness. As you are twisting, use your hand upon your left knee, drawing it or hugging it as you soften your body toward sitting position. When you draw your knee toward your chest, the thigh bone will literally release in the hip area. This presses against the piriformis and encourages it to release.

This twist will deepen when you draw your knee into your elbow, or place your upper arm near the outside of the knee. As you are pressing your knee against your arm for leverage, the pose will be more active in the area of the hip, and less effective in releasing the piriformis. If you have piriformis syndrome, don't twist deeply.

Video: https://www.youtube.com/watch?v=-yw48KAe_8M

The Piriformis Stretch

A half twist of the spine will stretch your piriformis mildly and encourage it to lengthen and release. The intensity may then be progressively increased. Don't stretch too aggressively, or it may bring on sciatic pain. Proceed slowly and carefully, adjusting the pose for minimal discomfort.

Preparing for the Spinal Twist

Sit at the corner of a folded-up blanket with knees bent and feet on your floor right in front of you. Next, put your right foot under the left knee and then around to the outside of the left hip. The right knee should be pointing forward. In a mild hip stretch, put your left foot down on the floor inside the right knee.

Lean onto the left lower pelvic ("sit") bone and balance your weight between your hips. This will begin the stretch. Keep yourself steady by holding onto your left knee with both hands. Inhale and feel the lengthening through your spine. If it feels too intense, or you feel pain, add to the padding beneath your hips to make the stretch more comfortable.

If you feel no stretch in your hip, pull your left knee gently across your body's midline toward your right chest, while you keep your sit bones grounded equally. Resist the thigh a bit against your pulling hands. This will keep the sit bone well-grounded, to increase the piriformis stretch.

Remain in this pose from 30 seconds to a minute or two. Repeat on your other side.

More stretches to fight sciatica

Hamstring Stretches

Hamstring stretches are important in sciatic pain relief, since tight hammies along with a tight piriformis may constrict the sciatic nerve. Sciatic pain that is caused by the tightening of hamstrings and the surrounding muscles commonly comes from activities like athletics, or driving for a long time, especially if your car seat encourages a rounded or slumped posture. If this is the case, take a break or rest stop and then use hamstring stretches.

Standing hamstring stretches

Place your right foot on a bench, chair or table. It should be at the level of your hips, or lower. Keep the leg straight with your toes and knees pointing up, and engage your quadriceps. If your knee becomes hyperextended or locked, protect it with an exercise band. Be sure that the hip of the raised leg isn't lifted, just releasing downward. The foot and leg should not turn outward.

Hold this pose for a few breaths, and repeat on the other side. If you want to stretch more deeply, and you're comfortable doing so, bend over your leg from the hip, with your quadriceps firm and your leg and spine straight.

To aid in the right hip descent, loop a belt around the top of your thigh, on the lifted leg and the foot of the leg still standing straight. Pull downward or tighten the belt to draw down the thigh bone. You can concentrate on the side where you experience more pain, or alternate legs. Hold the position for several breaths.

King Pigeon hip stretch

This is the strongest piriformis stretch. You will only be bringing yourself to the edge of your stretch so that you can hold it and breathe, allowing the piriformis to properly release. Begin on hands and knees. Then bring your right knee out to the right and forward. Your right foot should be forward as well, until the heel is aligned with your left hip. The shin should be at an angle of about 45 degrees. Keep the foot flexed, to afford your knee protection.

In stretching the right piriformis, lean forward with your upper body while tucking under your left toes. Walk or slide your left leg back straight, while you allow the right thigh to rotate passively out. Your hip will descend towards the floor. Maintain level hips and don't allow your pelvis to fall or turn to one side. If your right hip doesn't reach all the way to the floor, support it with a blanket.

Remain in this pose for at least several breaths and at most one minute. Experiment a bit by leaning forward with your upper body, over your shin, and try bringing your torso into a more upright position, which will vary the hip stretch.

If this pose is too difficult or intense for you, there is another variation. Place your right leg on a table top and then lean forward. Use your hands for balance and walk your left foot back.

Modified cow's face pose

This is an excellent example of a gentle, passive hip rotator stretch. Sitting on the floor, extend your legs forward. Bend the right knee, bringing your right leg across the left. Using your hand, draw the right foot close to the outer side of your left hip. Move the left foot across to the right. Use your hands resting on the floor, and wiggle and lift your hips until it stacks your knees. Your right knee will be above your left.

If you are seated on a blanket, or your left leg (the back of it) doesn't touch the floor, or if your left knee hurts or locks while stretching, roll up another blanket, placing it under the left knee for added support. Use your left hand to hold your right foot in place.

Breathe in and lengthen and lift through the spine to the top of your head. While you exhale, fold forward from the hip, and bring your chest down towards your knee. Keep your neck relaxed and long. Move like you are trying to bring your navel towards your knee. Keep your spine relaxed and extended.

You will likely feel more stretching on the outer side of the straightened leg, along the outer calf and hamstring. You may also feel a milder stretch within the right hip. Help your hamstrings to release by keeping your quadriceps engaged. To increase right hip stretch, turn your chest a bit to the right. Extend through the inner heel and big toe of the straight leg, so that your little toe side of the foot is drawn back a bit. This firms the outer shin.

Keep your toes pointing upward. If you are able, use your right hand to hold the outer side of your left foot. Do not pull back strongly, or you may jam your hip and outer knee. Hold this position from several regular breaths up to a minute or so. Then repeat the stretch on the other side.

Herbs that Help you Fight Sciatica

If you have sciatic pain, you can find relief in the stretching we have discussed, along with other exercise and position-changing. You may also turn to NSAIDs for the treatment of your pain. Over time, these over-the-counter drugs may become less effective, especially during flare-ups.

If you'd prefer not to use prescription pain medications due to side effects, you have alternatives. They're not known as widely as OTC drugs, since herbal medicine manufacturers cannot afford to advertise like big drug companies do. In addition, they don't receive as much attention from medical professionals as OTC and prescription drugs do. Still, many herbal choices have been proven to be effective against sciatic pain.

1. **Garlic**

   Garlic contains amazing properties as an anti-inflammatory, which makes it a natural treatment for sciatica pain. Use more garlic in your meal preparation, and consider using the cloves as a dietary supplement. A few raw cloves in the morning are quite helpful in fighting pain, and they boost your immune system, too.

2. **Saint John's Wort Oil**

   St. John's Wort is a flowering plant that has been used in medicine since the ancients discovered its effects, in Greece. It is effective in treating nerve pain. Its properties also include antioxidants, antibacterials, astringents and anti-inflammatories. It can help in the regeneration of nerve tissue and relieve sciatic pain.

3. Jamaican Dogwood

This comes from dogwood tree bark, and it is a powerful nerve pain relief substance. You can apply it in tincture form or as a supplement in capsules. If you are a pregnant or lactating woman, do not use Jamaican dogwood.

4. Turmeric

Turmeric is becoming more popular as an anti-inflammatory herb. It has a long-standing record in natural healing and health. Turmeric's anti-inflammatory properties help in reducing sciatic swelling and pain by lowering the body's inflammation-fueling enzymes. You can drink turmeric in tea, cook with it or apply it in a topical paste.

Conclusion

Within this article, we have given you practical information about what causes sciatic pain and how it is diagnosed. We've delved into the best ways to treat sciatic pain, from conventional medications and surgery to stretching, yoga and herbal medicines.

You've found out now that you don't have to suffer from sciatic pain on a continuous basis. With the ways we have described, you can fight back and win against the rigors of sciatic pain.

Be sure that you consult with your primary care physician or specialist before you try any of the ways we have suggested to fight sciatica. We wish you the best in recovering from sciatic pain.

www.ingramcontent.com/pod-product-compliance
Lightning Source LLC
Chambersburg PA
CBHW070245290526
45789CB00004B/1771